A PATIENT'S GUIDE TO CATARACT SURGERY

Normal and LASIK Reshaped Cornea

Kady Dash

ISBN: 9798481402505
ISBN: 9798465336567

Printed in the United States of America

Limit of Liability/Disclaimer of Warranty

While the publisher and author have used their best efforts in preparing this book, they make no representations or warranties with respect to the accuracy or completeness of the contents of this book and specifically disclaim any implied warranties of merchantability or fitness for a particular purpose. No warranty may be created or extended by sales representatives or written sales materials. The advice and strategies contained herein may not be suitable for your situation. You should consult with a professional when appropriate. Neither the publisher nor the author shall be liable for any loss of profit or any other commercial damages, including but not limited to special, incidental, consequential, personal, or other damages.

CONTENTS

*This book is dedicated to my mother, who
gave me vision and so so much more.*

Fact One: Cataract surgery is simple, painless and risk free ... the whole procedure is common, routine and nothing to worry about. Fact Two: Fact One applies only to cataracts on the eyes in somebody else's head.

AUTHOR: HELENE HANFF

PROLOGUE

Forty years ago, I had LASIK surgery, and I was happy with the results. I gave no thought to what would happen if, like most people, I should need cataract surgery in the future. I had the surgery within ten years of when it became available in the United States at Mass Eye and Ear Hospital in Boston, a top hospital dedicated to ophthalmology. Since I am in the first wave of people having cataract surgery after LASIK surgery, I hope that sharing my experience might be helpful to other people. I will share what people should do before needing cataract surgery if they have had LASIK surgery previously. This information is the core purpose of this book, as this information is not well known.

INTRODUCTION

This book will provide a step-by-step account of four cataract surgeries: Two surgeries my husband underwent and of my surgeries. Unlike me, my husband had 20/20 vision without undergoing LASIK surgery.

I will describe what happens before, during, and after cataract surgery in both situations. I will compare both procedures side by side, highlighting the differences between them. My goal is to provide insights that are only available from the patient's perspective to supplement the information you receive from the medical professionals.

Those contemplating getting the LASIK procedure will want to read this book to understand its implication for cataract surgery. After LASIK surgery, cataract surgery is not a simple surgery everyone thinks it to be.

BEFORE THE CATARACT SURGERY

My eye doctor told me for years that I had small cataracts that would need to be removed through surgery at some future point. When I asked, "How will I know when it is the right time?" He invariably replied, "You will know." Well, now I do know! And I will share with you the subtle signs that were not obvious to me initially.

Cataract surgery is one of the most common procedures, yet when I came face to face with it, there was a lot of information that came as a surprise to me. Though my husband and I had cataract surgeries the same year, our experiences were very different. He is a guy who has had a perfect vision for most of his life. I've been nearsighted since I was a child and had a LASIK procedure that corrected my vision to 20/20. Comparing our experiences gives an interesting contrast between "virgin" eyes and LASIK-repaired eyes.

My husband and I have the same eye doctor, so the surgical procedure and doctor's skills were the same. There are many similarities in our experiences, yet many differences even between the two eyes of the same person.

INITIAL SIGNS OF CATARACTS

Almost everyone requires cataract surgery at some point. My husband was the first of us to get a warning from the doctor that he had small cataracts in both eyes. A few years later, our eye doc gave me the same warning. The doctor monitored us for many years, saying that no corrective action was required.

Even though we got the warning separated by a few years and my husband is a few years older than I am, our cataracts developed to the point that they required surgery at about the same time. Our surgeries occurred six months apart. About a year before his surgery, my husband told me he felt uncomfortable driving at night. It was harder for him to see the turns and curves on the poorly lit roads. During one of my husband's eye doctor visits at about this time, the doctor said, "My friend, you are ready for the cataract surgery. Looking at your eyes, I would not want to ride in a car that you are driving."

Switching to my story, after my LASIK procedure, I always saw slight flaring around headlights at night and did not have a good nighttime vision. As my cataracts developed, these symptoms increased gradually. Because the changes were gradual, I did not recognize them until nighttime driving became almost impossible.

Because my nighttime vision has not been good for so many years, the first signs I noticed were not nighttime driving. My first warning sign was being bothered by what I thought were smudges on my computer reading glasses. For several months, I diligently scrubbed my computer glasses to try to remove the smudges. I finally realized that the smudges were not on the glasses but in my eyes!

HOW YOU WILL KNOW WHEN YOU NEED A CATARACT SURGERY

In a normal eye, the lens is clear. In an eye that has a cataract, the lens is cloudy. Seeing with an eye that has a cataract is like looking through a cellophane bag or a steamed-up window.

When you have a cataract, you become more sensitive to bright lights and glare. As my cataracts worsened through the years, I noticed a change in the appearance of oncoming car headlights. The flair around each headlight became bigger and bigger. Just prior to my surgery, I couldn't look directly at oncoming cars because the light blinded me. I couldn't see the road ahead of me and would find myself braking when I saw on-coming traffic as I could not see whether I needed to go straight or if there was a curve in the road. I knew braking was not safe, but continuing to drive while unable to see the road was also unsafe.

The two images below show how headlights looked to me with and without cataracts. The glare caused by the cataracts was particularly challenging after the rain when I had to contend with not just the headlights but also their reflection on the road.

Picture 1. Traffic as it would look to a person with normal vision.

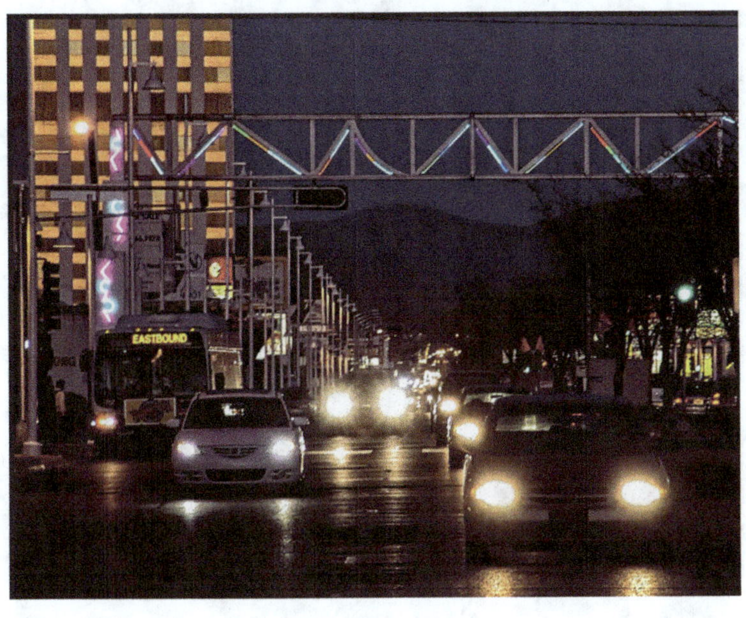

*Picture 2. Traffic as it would look to
a person with cataracts.*

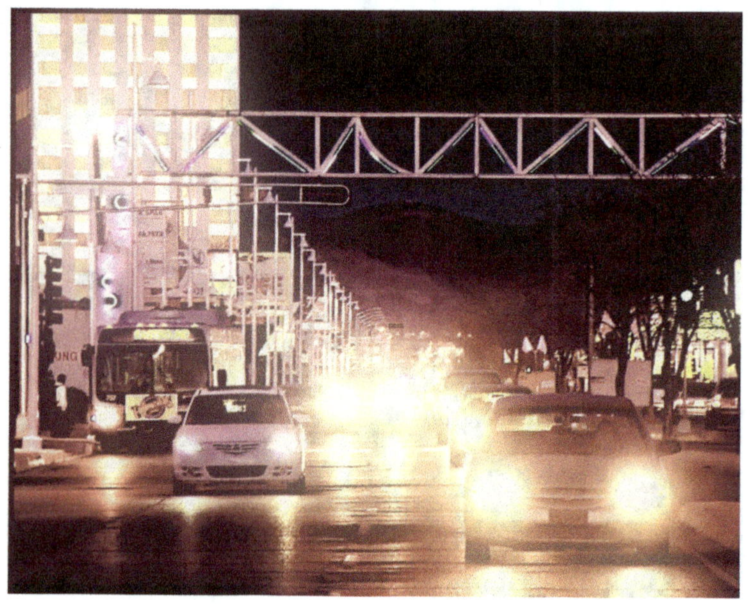

My husband's earliest symptoms were the inability to read a menu in the restaurant without a flashlight that he began carrying. The next symptom he felt was less confidence driving at night and not seeing the road well in the dark. The eye doctor said these are typical symptoms. Another symptom the doctor mentioned was painless blurred or double vision in one eye. (Blurred vision with pain is a different problem.) The doctor also mentioned fading or yellowing colors. This change is hard to notice because it is gradual. After I had a cataract removed in one eye and not the other, the difference became apparent, though.

The development of a cataract is usually age-related. Other causes are long-term use of certain medications, diabetes, overexposure to the sun, or an injury to the eye.

The cloudiness of the lens does not develop over the entire lens at once; if it develops first at the edge of the lens rather than the center, it is less of a hindrance. However, if left untreated, it will develop over the entire lens of the eye.

How quickly the cataract develops and grows is very individual. If it is due to normal aging, it usually takes years. When cataracts are caused by diabetes or medication, it might only take months.

As I mentioned earlier, the doctor told me for many years that I would know when I was ready for the cataract surgery. He did not tell me how I would know. Turns out what he meant was that doing everyday things, like driving at night, would become too difficult. And by "too difficult," I mean I felt I did not see well enough to drive safely.

BRIGHTNESS ACUITY TEST

A brightness acuity test can be used to confirm a need for cataracts. The brightness acuity test measures the degree of vision loss experienced in bright light. The tool my doctor used for the test looked like regular eyeglasses, except they had built-in lights around the frame that directed bright light into my eyes. Once the lights were shining into my eyes, the doctor asked me to read the standard eye chart. The vision in the right eye was reduced from 20/20 under normal light conditions to 20/40 with the bright light shining into my eye. Not terrible. However, during the left eye test, I could see only the white square of the eye chart and not any letters. Under normal light conditions, my vision in the left eye was 20/20. With the bright light shining into my eye, I was blind in my left eye. This test accurately simulated my sight at night with the car headlights shining into my eyes.

14

WHAT CATARACT SURGERY CORRECTS

During cataract surgery, the surgeon removes the cloudy lens from the eye and replaces it with an acrylic intraocular lens implant. The surgeon makes a very small incision, and the lens is inserted, rolled, or folded to fit through the tiny opening. Once inside, the lens unfolds to about a quarter of an inch in size. Side struts, called haptics, hold the implant in place. The incision is so small that stitches are not required. The lens implants become part of the eye. The lenses are stable, and they require no care or maintenance. I asked the doctor if they would last more than 30 years, and he said "yes."

Picture 3. How the lens is inserted into the eye.

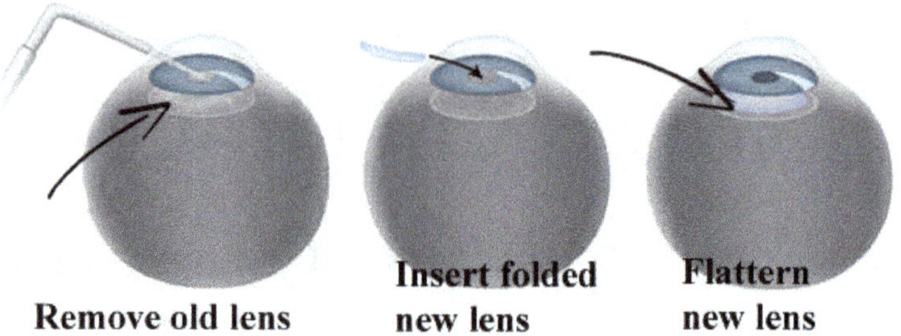

WHAT CATARACT SURGERY DOES NOT CORRECT

What does cataract surgery not correct? It does not fix floaters. Floaters are caused by debris floating in the vitreous humour, a watery substance in the eyeball between the lens and retina of the eye. Floaters are often caused by aging, although I was 18 years old when I first noticed mine. I was afraid they were a sign of something terrible happening, but the eye doctor reassured me they were harmless.

Cataract surgery also does not fix cornea scarring from LASIK. Scarring from LASIK often causes halos to be seen around lights, and a new lens will not fix that visual effect.

Picture 4. Structure of the eye.

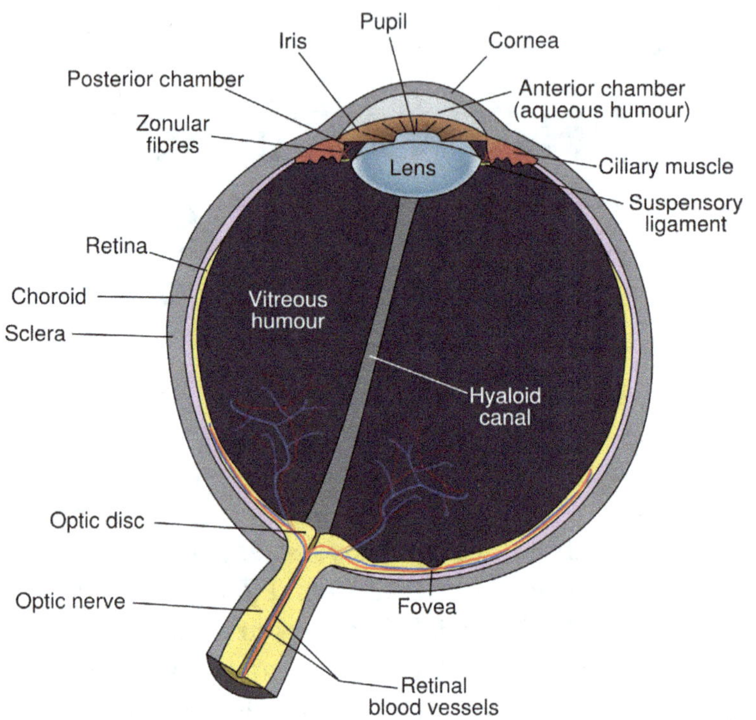

LENS OPTIONS

The doctor set up a consultation appointment prior to my surgery to review the procedure and the lens options. He described three options: mono-focal lenses, multi-focal lenses, and accommodating lenses. Our eye surgeon only uses the first two options, and I included his explanation of the three options and why he stopped using accommodating lenses in this chapter. The three lens options exist for people who have not undergone LASIK surgery in the past. LASIK introduces additional challenges in finding the correct power and lens shape due to the re-shaped cornea. To improve the chances of a good outcome, my doctor recommended that I only consider mono-focal lenses. His recommendation for my husband was to use multi-focal lenses.

Other than having LASIK surgery, my doctor said I had no high-risk conditions. I had no other eye surgeries, eye trauma, diabetes, or eye abnormalities. My cataract was not dense, my lacrimal duct (the duct that conducts tears) was normal. The cataract in my left eye was more noticeable to me than the cataract in the right eye because of its position in the center of my vision. The doctor has warned me that in his experience, patients who had LASIK surgery are harder to fit with a perfect lens. My prior LASIK surgery was the only reason why he recommended a mono-vision lens.

Single-focus lens

A single-focus lens, also referred to as an intraocular lens (IOL) or mono-focal IOL, has a fixed focal point. These lenses are optimized either for distance or reading vision and typically require eyeglasses. A lens optimized for distance requires reading glasses. A lens optimized for reading requires glasses for distance. You can expect to see well at all distances with a single-focus lens used with the appropriate bifocal (or trifocal) eyeglasses.

An additional strategy using single-focus lenses to give clear vision both near and far without glasses is called mono-vision. This technique uses a distance-optimized lens in one eye and a reading-optimized lens in the other. Not everyone is comfortable with this difference in focus, but many people find they adapt well to mono-focus lenses. If you are interested in this option, try it out for a few weeks using contact lenses before having cataract surgery.

Single-focus lenses are fully covered by insurance, and you typically pay only a doctor visit co-pay out of pocket.

Multi-focus lens

A multi-focus lens (also referred to as a multifocal IOL) has different focus zones that allow a wide range of vision and decreased dependence on eyeglasses. Since this type of lens works by dividing the light that enters the eye, it can produce glare and halos at night in some percentage of patients. My doctor said that five out of 1000 patients complain about these issues. My husband received a multi-focus lens and does not see halos or glare.

Multi-focus lenses are not fully covered by insurance.

Accommodating-focus lens

An accommodating-focus lens responds to contracting and loosening of the ciliary muscles. It moves within the eye to accommodate the entire range of vision. The ciliary muscle changes the shape of the synthetic lens, just as it did the natural lens when it was still flexible before the onset of age-related presbyopia. Though a patient's vision will improve immediately after implantation of this type of lens, it can take up to a year for the ciliary muscle to adjust to the new lens for optimal vision. While the person gets used to the lens, the clarity of the vision varies. My doctor does not perform surgery with this type of lens due to the high number of patients who report dissatisfaction with the results.

As with any surgery, there are risks; the worst is blindness, but this complication is rare.

Astigmatism

Astigmatism is an uneven curvature of the eye's cornea or lens. A normal eye is shaped like a basketball. An eye with astigmatism is shaped like an American football. When the cornea and lens are curved equally in all directions (the basketball case), the light rays focus sharply onto the retina at the back of your eye. If the cornea or lens is curved unevenly (the football case), light rays are not refracted perfectly to focus in one spot. This imperfect focus is the refractive error caused by astigmatism. Cataract surgery can correct this refractive error in several ways.

The first option is a laser vision correction procedure called Photorefractive Keratectomy (PRK) after implantation of a multi-focus or a single-focus lens if astigmatism or other refractive problem remains after the surgery. PRK is not covered by insurance, and if we had had the procedure, the cost would have been $2,500 per eye for a total of $5,000. Neither of us selected this option; I opted for a single-focus toric lens to correct my slight astigmatism.

Toric lens variation is available in both single-focus and multi-focus lenses. Toric lenses compensate for the different curvature of the cornea in the eye caused by astigmatism. The shape of toric lenses creates different focusing powers on the vertical and horizontal orientations. The refractive strength increases or decreases gradually around the lens. Toric lenses have a middle axis, like the Earth's equator, that keeps your line of vision clear. Since toric lenses have a particular orientation, they need to be placed into your eye in the correct way.

PREPARATION FOR THE SURGERY

The eye doctor required each patient to get a standard pre-operative physical exam from the primary care physician. The main part of this exam involves performing an EKG to ensure that the patient will not have heart problems during the surgery. The doctor's pre-surgery report is valid for only 30 days, so the primary care visit must be coordinated with the cataract surgery date. A nurse practitioner can perform the exam instead of the physician, if necessary.

A few weeks before surgery, the surgeon performed an A- scan that precisely measured and mapped the eye. The scan helped the doctor determine the correct power for the implanted lens before the surgery.

Our surgeries were performed on each eye at separate times. My husband, who had 20/20 vision and no prior LASIK surgery, was scheduled to do each eye 30 days apart. The dominant eye was done first.

In my case, the eye with the more severe cataract was done first. It was my non-dominant eye. My second eye surgery was also scheduled 30 days later, but complications from the surgery on the first eye caused it to be postponed indefinitely. The details of the complications are described later in the book.

Four days before the first surgery, my husband and I were required to treat the eye by applying a daily drop of the medication Voltaren (generic name Diclofenac sodium). The last dose of the medication was done the morning of the surgery.

LASIK SURGERY RECORDS

For anyone who has had LASIK surgery, it is vital to obtain the records from the hospital where the surgery was done. The most important information is the A-scan that was performed before the LASIK surgery, which contains information about the cornea shape before it was changed by LASIK. This information is an important part of selecting the correct lens during cataract surgery.

Typically, the hospital is obligated to keep these records for only 10 or 15 years. So it is imperative to get a copy of this information as soon as the LASIK surgery is done so that it'll be available when you need cataract surgery years down the road.

My LASIK surgery was not done by my regular ophthalmologist, so it was not part of my regular record. Instead, I had the surgery done at a Boston eye and ear hospital that specialized in the procedure. My regular ophthalmologist at the time never suggested that I get a copy of the records, and I did not think of it myself. Fortunately, when I switched to my current doctor, it was one of the first things he told me to do. At the time, it had been almost 15 years since my LASIK surgery, and I was fortunate that they still had my records. I spoke with them on the phone, and shortly after I completed the HIPA paperwork, a thick stack of papers and scans was in my hands.

This advice might be the most critical piece of information in this book: Make sure you have a copy of your LASIK surgery records.

BEFORE THE FIRST SURGERY, THE NORMAL CORNEA

My husband's cataract surgery was scheduled for 8 A.M. on a surgical floor of a hospital. My husband was not allowed to drive that day, so I was chauffeuring him around. On the day of surgery, he was instructed to avoid all food, vitamins, supplements, and drinks except for a small amount of clear water and any necessary prescription medications. This helps to ensure an empty stomach for the surgery and avoids complications with anesthesia.

In the hospital, he changed into a hospital gown; they allowed him to keep his underwear, but everything else had to go. The nurses inserted an IV into his arm but did not start it. They put a blue dot on his forehead above the eye to be operated on.

As soon as the IV was inserted, the nurses led me to join him in the pre-op room so he would have company. The hospital staff thought it would be relaxing to have a family member to talk to while he waited for the procedure.

For an hour before surgery, the nurses put various eye drops into his eye every 10 minutes. Some eye drops were painless; some burned a little. Overall, it was completely tolerable. The last two sets of the drops were a numbing gel. After the first application of the gel, he no longer could tell if they were putting drops into his eye. He kept asking, "Did you miss it?" They assured him it was a good sign that he could not feel the drops.

During this period, both the anesthesiologist and the surgeon visited the room. The anesthesiologist checked if he had had any food and if he had indigestion. The doctor said he would have given him Prilosec if he had indigestion. The surgeon just said hello. Every nurse and every doctor who visited asked his name, date of birth, and what procedure he was undergoing. It was reassuring!

BEFORE THE FIRST SURGERY, THE LASIK RESHAPED CORNEA

My pre-op routine was similar. I knew what to expect from my husband's procedure six months earlier. I recall feeling very relaxed from the Valium they gave me while waiting for the procedure to start.

SURGERY, THE NORMAL CORNEA

At 9:15 am, my husband's right eye was prepped for surgery. The nurses started the IV with an anesthetic in it. Sedation was very light; the nurses jokingly described it as the equivalent of two shots of martinis. My husband was awake, but his body was relaxed, and he was very mellow. The doctor only anesthetized the eye using the gel. He said that some surgeons use an injection under the eye, but he finds that his patients heal faster with just the gel.

My husband was wheeled into an operating room and the nurses attached a device that kept his eye opened and prevented him from blinking. His left eye was covered by a white cloth, so he could not see what was going on. The procedure itself lasted 30 minutes. He said he did not feel a thing, no pain, no pressure, nothing. During the procedure, he saw

LED lights out of the eye being operated on, but he did not know what they were. He did not see the surgeon.

When the procedure was over, the doctor asked him to focus on a red dot. And then they rolled him into the post-op room.

*Picture 5. Speculum that keeps the
eye open during surgery.*

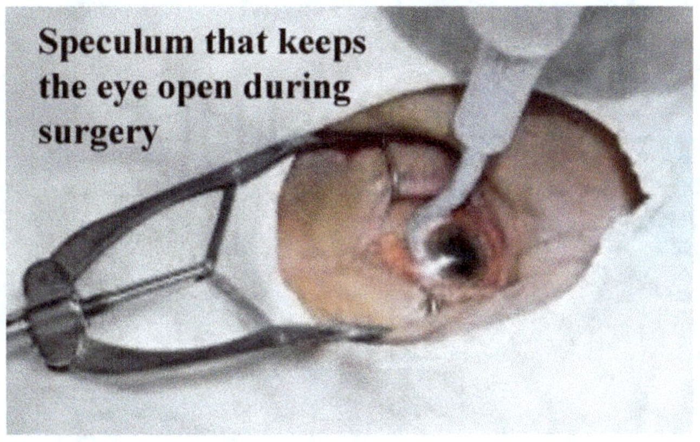

SURGERY, THE LASIK RESHAPED CORNEA

My LASIK surgeries had reshaped the corneas of my eyes, which affected the calculations for finding the best fit for a replacement lens. Besides using the old A-scans, my surgeon used an extra procedure called intraoperative Optiwave Refractive Analysis (ORA) technology to make the calculations more accurate, which he would not use for the normal cornea. The ORA is attached to the surgical microscope and uses intraoperative wavefront aberrometry to measure the eye's refractive power once the cataract is removed. This on-demand power calculation is then used to ensure proper implant power, lens placement, and determination of the magnitude and direction of astigmatism. ORA performs 40 different calculations to measure the eye's refractive power to determine the correction required by the intraocular lens implant. These measurements enable the surgeon to compensate for inaccuracies the LASIK reshaped cornea introduces. ORA is helpful for patients who have had previous refractive surgery, such as LASIK, PRK, or RK, as well as people with extreme near or far-sightedness, or higher amounts of astigmatism. ORA technology is not covered by insurance. My doctor charged $1000 per eye for its use.

The surgery was painless. I was fully awake, hearing clicks and whirls of the machinery and conversations between the surgeon and medical staff. My eyelids were held open by a device to prevent blinking. Because of the numbing drops in the eye, none of it felt unpleasant.

AFTER THE FIRST SURGERY, BOTH CORNEAS

My husband stayed in the post-op room for about 30 minutes so he could be observed for any side effects. Then they told him to get dressed and wheeled him out in a wheelchair to the front entrance. While he was getting dressed, a nurse told me I should get my car and drive to the front entrance. The time was 10:30 am, two and a half hours after we arrived.

The patient said he felt fine. He was not groggy or in pain. However, the vision out of the operated eye was fuzzy. The doctor explained that the vision was affected by the goopy eye drops and dilation. He said to expect the fuzzy vision to last until the next day.

At 3:00 pm, I drove my husband to the doctor's office

for a post-surgical check. The nurses checked his eye pressure and the doctor looked at his eye and told him everything looked good. His next appointment for another evaluation was scheduled in 10 days.

My schedule and overall experience on the day of the first surgery were similar.

POST-SURGERY EYE DROP REGIMEN, BOTH CORNEAS

After the surgery, both of us had a rigorous eye drop regimen for six weeks. One eye drop was taken once a day, two others three times a day, and over-the-counter artificial tears as needed, at least three times a day. The doctor gave each of us a chart to mark off the eye drops we took each day, to track the medication taken every day. We both wore a plastic eye patch taped to the face during the night to prevent accidental pokes by a pillow.

PROGRESS REPORTS, NORMAL CORNEA

My husband received multi-focus lenses, which allowed him to see in the distance and to read without glasses.

Immediately after the surgery, normal cornea

Immediately after my husband's surgery, both distance and reading vision were fuzzy.

Eight hours after surgery, normal cornea

Eight hours after the surgery, the distance vision became reasonably clear. My husband could read a book 12 inches away but reported that the text 10 inches away was fuzzy. However, at 12 inches, the operated eye was more clear than the non-operated eye at the same distance.

The wall paint my husband previously thought was off-white looked whiter. Closing one eye at a time, he could tell the difference between the dingy off-white seen with the non-operated eye and the near-total white seen with the surgically repaired eye. The TV looked much brighter and more clear. He joked that he felt like he bought a new, better TV.

Ten hours after surgery, normal cornea

Ten hours after the surgery, my husband reported the text at 10 inches was still fuzzy, but that if he used his old reading glasses, the text at 10 inches was crystal clear.

He tested his computer vision, looking at the 30-inch computer monitor. He could see all parts of the screen in focus. This was a much better experience than the eyeglasses with progressive lenses, where you can tell that glasses have bands with a different focus. When I look at a large computer screen with computer glasses that use progressive lenses, I need to keep adjusting the position of my head to see different portions of the screen clearly. My husband said that he did not have to move his head to find the best focus area; the focus felt very natural. The multi-focus lenses felt more natural than the progressive lenses in eyeglasses.

Four days after surgery, normal cornea

My husband's long-distance vision with the operated eye was very good almost from the outset. Four days after the surgery, that had not changed. The middle distance (for example, looking at the computer screen) became crisp the next day after surgery. He stopped using computer glasses. The entire 30-inch area of his large monitor appeared in focus.

Four days after the surgery, he could read a book and a paper newspaper without eyeglasses. The text looked a little fuzzy when looking with each eye individually, although the vision was better with the operated eye. However, when he looked at the book or the newspaper with both eyes, he could see the text clearly without eyeglasses. The brain was able to triangulate two somewhat fuzzy images into a combined clear image.

His vision kept changing every day, so he was unsure if vision quality on a given day reflected the final surgery results or if his vision would continue to improve.

One week after the surgery, normal cornea

A week after surgery, the vision in the operated eye

was crisp at all distances. The colors were bright and clear. After cataract surgery, some people have light sensitivity, but my husband reported that the bright lights or sun reflections did not bother him. He is the type of person that does not like wearing sunglasses and having cataract surgery did not force him to change his habits.

PROGRESS REPORTS, LASIK RESHAPED CORNEA

I had a toric single-focus lens implanted into my left eye. The doctor thought the single-focus lens would provide the best chances for a successful outcome given the complications introduced by LASIK surgery.

Immediately after the surgery, LASIK reshaped cornea

Immediately after the surgery, my vision was bad. But I was not worried because I knew from my husband's experience that the vision would not be good from the dilation and the protective gel covering the eyeball.

Eight hours after surgery, LASIK reshaped cornea

This is where my story diverges from that of my husband. Eight hours after the surgery, my vision continued to be bad. When I looked at the computer screen, I saw the screen but no text on the screen. I felt pain in the eye. My eye looked swollen. I took over-the-counter pain medication (Nuprin), and that helped. During the follow-up appointment on the day of the surgery, the doctor told me to give it some more time.

Ten hours after surgery, LASIK reshaped cornea

The pain subsided, but the vision was still very unclear.

Ten days after surgery, LASIK reshaped cornea

After ten days, I could see the text on the computer screen, but my distance vision was very poor. The doctor tested my eyes during the ten-day follow-up and confirmed that I could not see anything on the eye chart, even the top line.

The doctor gave me three options:
- PRK surgery six months down the line to correct distance vision.
- Trifocal glasses for distance vision, medium (computer screen) distance, and close-up (reading) distance.
- Re-doing the cataract surgery.

The situation was nerve-wracking because test glasses did not correct my vision. The doctor told me the test glasses didn't correct my vision yet because my cornea was still swollen. A cornea reshaped by LASIK is more sensitive and reacts by swelling more than a normal cornea. He thought repeating the cataract surgery would give me the best outcome. I opted for repeat cataract surgery.

The longer you wait for repeat surgery, the stronger the implant attaches to the eye and the harder it becomes to remove. So the repeat cataract surgery had to be done right away.

THE SECOND SURGERY, NORMAL CORNEA

My husband's second eye surgery itself was quite similar to the first. Before the surgery, I had a chance to ask the surgeon if my husband would stay awake throughout the procedure, and the doctor confirmed that he would. The sedation only relaxes the patient; it does not put the patient out.

As he was discharged from the hospital, the staff told him to contact the doctor immediately if he saw flashing lights or was in significant pain. Just like after the first eye surgery, he saw the doctor six hours after the surgery in the doctor's office. His next appointment was ten days later.

SECOND SURGERY (THE RE-DO), LASIK RESHAPED CORNEA

When the lens is inserted into the eye, it is rolled up and inserted through a small opening. When it is in place, it unfurls and flattens to its full size. It is not possible to remove the unfurled lens through the same opening used to insert it. The surgeon had two options to remove the lens: cut it into small pieces while in my eye and remove it piece by piece or enlarge the opening and remove it in one piece. The surgeon chose to enlarge the opening because it was a less risky procedure. A larger opening required a stitch to close it, which caused a higher degree of post-surgery pain.

48

PROGRESS REPORTS, NORMAL CORNEA

Even though my husband's second surgery felt the same as the first, the recovery immediately after the second surgery was different.

The day of the second surgery, normal cornea

My husband's left eye felt more irritated than the right eye after the first surgery. During the afternoon follow-up appointment on the day of the surgery, the doctor said that the left eye was slightly swollen. He said it was not something to worry about, that it was not unusual, and the swelling should go down shortly. The eye was dilated and covered with a special goop to protect it during the first day, so it was impossible to assess the vision in the eye right away.

By the end of the first day after the first eye surgery, the right eye could focus on the items at a long distance. This was not the case with his left eye.

The day after the second surgery, normal cornea

The blurriness at all distances continued throughout the second day. With the first surgically-repaired eye closed, my husband could read the headlines in the newspaper but not the text of the articles. The blurriness was not helped by reading glasses; the old reading glasses made things worse. Despite the blurriness in the second eye, my husband was able to work on the computer the same long hours as he usually did, with the first eye doing all the work.

The irritation in the second eye subsided in the middle of the day, but came back in the evening. My husband no longer described it as an irritation but as pain. He had been using more teardrops than with the first eye.

Similar to after the first surgery, he needed to wear an eye patch to prevent poking himself in the eye during the night. The patch needed to be worn for a week.

Four days after the second surgery, normal cornea

Four days after the surgery, the second eye was no longer in pain, and the vision was good at all distances, although not as good as the first eye.

Ten days after the second surgery, normal cornea

A week after surgery, the vision in the newly-operated eye was crisp at all distances. My husband experienced no reflections, halos, or sensitivity to the sun.

Both eyes together and separately tested better than 20/20 on the vision test during a ten-day follow-up visit.

PROGRESS REPORTS, LASIK RESHAPED CORNEA

Immediately after the re-do surgery, LASIK reshaped cornea

Right after the surgery, my eye was swollen and covered. It was also dilated and covered with a protective gel, so even if it were not covered, I would not be able to assess my vision.

The day after the re-do surgery, LASIK reshaped cornea

The day after the surgery, I could see only black and white shapes, no details. The pain in the eye was significant, but eye drops and over-the-counter pain medicine made it tolerable.

Two days after the re-do surgery, LASIK reshaped cornea

After the two days, the pain in the eye was better. While I could see more than just shapes, my vision was still terrible.

After the first surgery, I returned to work the day after the surgery. It was distracting not to see with both eyes, but I managed with the right eye doing all the work. After the second surgery, I had to take a couple of days off. The combination of pain and the constant need for lubricating eye drops to soothe the irritation made working on the computer difficult.

During a follow-up visit after two days, the doctor told me that my vision was affected by the swollen cornea. He proved it to me by making me look at the eye chart with special glasses with pinholes in them. With these glasses on, I could see the two top lines on the eye chart.

Pinhole glasses are eyeglasses with lenses that have a grid of tiny holes. These glasses help the eyes focus by shielding the vision from indirect rays of light. By letting less light into your eye, less of the vision was distorted by the swollen cornea, and I could see more clearly. Pinhole glasses are also called stenopeic glasses.

My vision after the second surgery was better than after the first surgery. And with stenopeic eyeglasses, I felt hopeful that I would not be blind in the left eye.

Ten days after the re-do surgery, LASIK reshaped cornea

Ten days after the surgery, I had occasional glimpses of clear vision. They would come and go during the day. I primarily relied on the non-operated eye for working and driving.

Six-month after the re-do surgery, LASIK reshaped cornea

The periods of clear vision continued to increase over the next six months until, at the six-month check-up, I had 20/20 distance vision in the repaired eye. I still needed reading glasses for reading (+2.00) and computer glasses for using a computer (+1.00). However, the need for glasses was expected with the single-focus lens.

PUNCTAL PLUGS

I noticed an increased dryness in my eye after the cataract surgery. My ophthalmologist suggested I try punctal plugs. Punctal plugs prevent rapid draining of the tears through your nasolacrimal tear duct. The fact that the drainage is blocked keeps a protective tear film on the eye for a longer time.

TYPES OF PLUGS

The plugs are shaped like cylinders. Their size ranges from 0.2mm to over 1mm in width and 3 mm in length.

There are several types of punctal plugs; some are made of collagen, and others are made of silicone. They are inserted into the puncta of the eyelid. The puncta are the drainage openings of the eyelid, where tears drain down into the nasolacrimal duct. If the puncta are closed by the plugs, tears do not flow out of the eyes and stay in the eyes for longer.

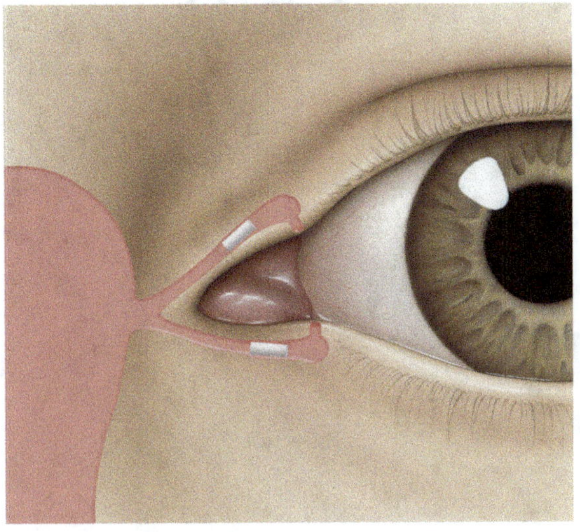

Collagen plugs placement.

Collagen plugs are not permanent; they typically last three months before they dissolve naturally in the body. That means they would need to be replaced regularly to provide continued relief. The benefit of dissolvable plugs is that they offer no risk of infection or inflammation. In addition, they are completely invisible as they are embedded below the puncta opening.

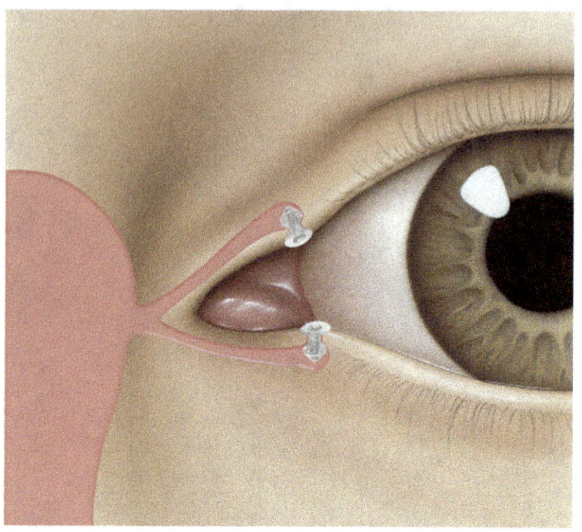

Silicone plugs placement.

Silicone plugs can last for years. They typically sit on top of the puncta, so they are visible as white dots in the corners of the eyes. They could be removed with tweezers if needed. Silicone plugs tend to have a higher infection rate than collagen plugs. If an infection occurs, the silicone plugs need to be taken out until the infection is treated and gone. The plugs can fall out (especially if you rub your eyelids) or fall into the tear duct. If these plugs slip into the inside of your tear duct, they can be removed either by irrigation or surgery.

The third type of plug is the intracanalicular plug. These plugs are inserted into the canalicular horizontally. These plugs are inserted deeper into the duct than punctal plugs and cannot be seen after insertion. They cannot be removed in the way punctal plugs can, though sometimes they may be flushed out with irrigation. In other cases, surgery might be necessary to remove them. These plugs are mostly made of silicone, although some newer materials used are acrylic polymer and hydrogel. Intracanalicular plugs are used less frequently than punctal plugs.

If a patient is a frequent eye rubber or has a large puncta, which will require a large plug, collagen plugs are a better option.

SILICONE PLUGS TRIAL AND ERROR

I tried silicone plugs and found them very uncomfortable. I was so uncomfortable that I had to have them removed after two days of pain. My left eye and my right eye have different size puncta openings. The left eye that gets drier has a much larger punctum. Thus, the silicone plug in the left eye was significantly bigger than the right one. The right eye plug looked like a little white dot, whereas the left eye plug looked like a little white ball. I could feel the silicone plugs, and they irritated my eyes. I could not tolerate them for more than a few days.

Next, the doctor suggested I try collagen plugs. The collagen plugs were internal and did not irritate my eyes. I sensed their presence for about a day, but after a day, I stopped noticing them.

Collagen plugs were more expensive; they cost $450 per eye ($675 for both eyes). My insurance covered them at 80% once the deductible was met. Because they dissolved, the expense was recurring four times a year. Silicone plugs are less expensive, as they usually do not need to be reinserted.

THE PUNCTAL PLUG INSERTION PROCEDURE

I felt apprehensive on the day of the first procedure, but it turned out to be quick and painless. Punctal plug insertion was done on an outpatient basis in the doctor's office, in the same chair where he does regular eye exams. The doctor selected the size of the plug for my left eye, put some numbing drops into my eye, and inserted the plug into the tear duct using small forceps. For a narrow tear duct, the doctor would have needed to use an instrument called a lacrimal dilator to open the tear duct so that the plug could fit in, but my eye did not require this instrument.

The silicone plug sits on top of the tear duct opening in the corner of the eye, whereas the collagen plug has to be inserted further into the puncta. Both procedures took only a few minutes and were not painful.

On the first day after the collagen plug procedure, I noticed a slight pressure in the eyelid, but it was not painful. I did not experience any discomfort around the inner corner of my eye. The next day, my eyes felt normal. For me, the collagen plugs were a much better experience than the silicone plugs.

WHEN SHOULD PLUGS START WORKING?

I thought I would see the improvement instantly because the tear duct was closed. However, my doctor surprised me by saying it may take as long as one month to notice an improvement in eye dryness. Fortunately, I noticed the change pretty quickly, although it was not dramatic. My eye felt slightly less dry throughout the day, but the morning dryness was still significant. Even a month later, the morning dryness remained a problem.

Before I had the plug inserted, I wondered if my eyes would often brim with tears, and it would look like I was crying. But this fear was unfounded; I never had so many tears that they did not drain comfortably. Of course, the experience varies from person to person; this was how the plugs worked for me.

REMOVING PUNCTAL PLUGS

How tear duct plugs are removed depends on the plug type. Collagen plugs cannot be removed, but they dissolve on their own in several months. Silicone punctal plugs sit closer to the eyelid's surface, and a doctor can remove them with forceps. My silicone plugs were removed after several days, and the procedure was painless. Intracanalicular plugs sit deeper in the duct and require surgery for removal.

While plugs are a common treatment for dry eyes, it is an invasive treatment and carries risks, such as infections. It is important to discuss with your optometrist or ophthalmologist your treatment options and the relative risks.

FINAL RESULTS

A bit down the road from our cataract surgeries, our vision is still excellent. We both still test as 20/20 vision. Sometimes when we drive, we compete over who can read a sign or license plate the farthest away. The cataract in my right eye is not as bad as the one in my left eye had been at the time I had the surgery. I have not done the second cataract surgery yet. The first experience was rather traumatic and made me want to wait to do the second surgery until it is absolutely necessary. As my doctor said, "You will know when you will need it." And now I do. And I hope after reading this book, so will you.

EPILOGUE

Any time someone touches your eyes, it is frightening. Any time you have surgery, there is a reason to be concerned. However, cataract surgery is a very common procedure. As long as you go to a surgeon who has done many of these surgeries, the doctor will know how to handle any problem. Even though my experience was nerve-wracking, I got through it successfully, and I am happy with the outcome.

THANK YOU

Thank you for taking the time to read this book and to hear what I felt was important to share, especially with those who have had LASIK surgery. Make sure you have your surgery records for the time when you will need the cataract surgery.

If you found this book helpful, please leave a review to let other potential readers know you found some value in reading this book.

ACKNOWLEDGEMENT

This book would not be possible without my husband, who patiently shared everything he saw and felt during his surgeries. Thank you!

A huge thank you to my editors, who helped me bring this book to life. Young H. D. Kim, your keen insight combined with encouraging words helped bring this effort to the finish line. Kendra, thank you for making sure I wrote what I meant; I meant what I wrote. Thank you for always being so helpful and supportive. Matt, you always know how to find just the right word.

BOOKS BY THIS AUTHOR

Back Surgery Step By Step Recovery Guide: What Your Doctor Can't Tell You

Are you facing back surgery? This book will supplement the medical information provided by your doctor. Be prepared to have a faster and easier recovery from back surgery. I know, I've been through it. Learn about:

ITEMS to bring to the hospital and rehabilitation facility

16 mobility tools that will make rehabilitation easier

11 physical therapy exercises that ARE most effective for recovery

A realistic expectation of pain and limitations during recovery

How To Find Care For Your Elderly Parent: A Guide To Selecting Assisted Living And Nursing Home, Plus What To

Do When The Money Runs Out

Are you worried about taking care of your elderly parents? Do you know how to select the best facility for their needs and financial situation? Kady Dash shares her experiences of what you must know before choosing a place for mom or dad.

In this book you will learn:

• What eighty questions to ask before selecting a facility
• Legal advice Kady got about signing forms, including what not to sign
• What to do when the savings to pay for room and board run out
• Clarifications of questions on Medicaid forms
• Medicaid's unwritten rules, including deadlines that are not the final ones
• Specific additional information requests from the caseworker
• Concise tips that will save you money
• Links to useful websites and vital online forms

The author shares the experience she gained during a two-year journey of moving her mother from independent living to assisted living and then to a nursing home. She details the step-by-step process of what to do when the money to pay for the facilities ran out. Kady describes the obstacles she had to overcome so you can learn from her mistakes instead of your own.

It is easy to feel overwhelmed trying to make the best choices for your parent. This book is specific and detailed. It is the no-nonsense helping hand every caregiver needs.

Heal Your Shoulder: Rotator Cuff Rehabilitation

Do you work with a computer and have shoulder pain? You don't have to be an athlete to get a rotator cuff injury! A year ago, I was barely able to move my mouse without crumbling in pain. After several months of physical therapy and finding a substitute for in-person massage of my aching shoulder, I am back to feeling healthy and normal.
In this book, I share nine exercises and the substitute for the in-person massage that healed my shoulder.

Show Some Spine: The Most Effective Physical Therapy Exercises For A Strong Back

I spent many months doing supervised physical therapy exercises for lower back pain. This book is a collection of exercises and instructions that I found to be most effective in my rehabilitation. I add other exercises for variety but this core set of exercises always remains part of my routine. In our busy lives sometimes it is hard to find time to exercise. If you only have a few minutes a day to exercise "Show Some Spine" and make these ten exercises part of your day. Your back will thank you!

Eyelift Surgery And Recovery Diary: Ptosis, Eyelifts, Punctal Plugs, And Dry Eyes

Get a patient's perspective on eyelift surgery. Your surgeon will cover the technical aspects of the surgery, but only another patient's first-hand account can prepare you for what to expect day-to-day.

"Eyelift surgery and recovery diary" covers both drooping eye (ptosis) correction and regular eyelift surgery. Would you be able to work the day after the surgery? Would you get black eyes? When would you be comfortable going out in public? What items do you need to buy to aid the recovery?

Learn what to expect after the surgery and see the healing process through daily photos. Kady Dash also includes anatomical charts and medical details but makes them easy to understand by non-medical professionals.

This book is detailed and provides a mix of objective

advice and personal experience to give a good idea about the entire process, starting before the surgery through ten months after the surgery, so there will be no surprises. Anyone considering eyelift surgery would benefit from reading this guide.

PRAISE FOR AUTHOR

Her research is methodical, and she includes incredibly handy product reference links throughout the book. Everything from reacher-grabbers to personal hygiene items are discussed frankly, along with real-user feedback. ... I wish I had read this book before my surgery. This is a heartfelt reference written by someone who is reaching out to offer help to others, knowing that this type of thing is and can be scary - especially if you're on your own.

- JOHN M. VIZCARRA ABOUT "BACK SURGERY STEP BY STEP RECOVERY GUIDE"

Step by Step is a helpful guide for anyone who is about to undergo surgery. The book focuses on back surgery but it's applicable to any sort of major surgery that involves a hospital stay or a stint in a rehab facility. The book is not about the medical procedure, it's purpose is to help the patient's preparation so that unpleasantness of the whole process is minimized.

The author covers all the mistakes or trip-ups that can hinder your progress. This is a great list of "don't repeat these mistakes" recommendations that are useful.
-The best part of the book is the list of questions to ask—these provide double the benefit: you know what to ask, and you learn what issues can arise at the same time.
-A close second (if not a tie) is the list of forms you will need. Man, does that save time.

There is so much that makes this book easy to recommend. Most importantly for me was the author's generosity in emailing a spreadsheet of the essential questions to ask when looking for a care facility. This was hugely helpful for me in breaking through the inertia of having to take on such a daunting task. This alone was a great return on investment. Kady has done a tremendous job of capturing all the learning needed from her own journey and made it available for those who face the journey of placing a loved one in a care facility.

- NANCY A. FISCHER ABOUT "HOW TO FIND CARE FOR YOUR ELDERLY PARENT"

As a veteran and an expert in physical fitness who overcame both severe neck and back pains myself, I can tell the exercises introduced in this book are really helpful if employed correctly and consistently with patience; it takes time until the pain goes away since the irritation in nerve branches and nerve endings caused by any damaged disc in spine doesn't go away for a while.

- YOUNG KIM ABOUT "SHOW SOME SPINE"

One of the many reasons this little book is so valuable is the manner in which Kady relates her own experiences – including the diagnostic procedures of Xray and ultrasound by an orthopedic physician – and her attention to anatomic detail both in words and in excellent illustrations makes this guide a learning experience. She discusses injectable cortisone and the response and then enters into an informative discussion of her physical therapy. Using that background information she then presents the nine exercises (and equipment –resistance bands, heat/cold therapy, massage) that allow the reader to utilize her well-informed, self-care return to normalcy!